I0442119

THE HICCUPS TRICK

THE DEFINITIVE CURE FOR HICCUPS

GARETH FORMAN

ISBN: 1500781533
ISBN-13: 978-1500781538

DEDICATION

This book is dedicated to my wife, Sarah, for her
continued support in all my projects

.

CONTENTS

GARETH FORMAN

1 MY INSPIRATION FOR WRITING THIS BOOK

For years I was a regular sufferer of hiccups. Not that I had any diagnosed disorder that caused me to experience hiccups with any more severity than the next person; I simply seemed to get them more often than most. Sometimes they would be gone within a few minutes. On other occasions, they could last several hours.

Hiccups are a somewhat strange phenomenon, something that can even be a slight source of amusement, at least at first (and particularly when it's not *you* who's experiencing them!). Sometimes they can occur spontaneously, for no obvious reason; other times the reason is more obvious (following heavy intake of alcohol, for example!).

Following the initial amusement, however, they can quickly become annoying, and even quite painful; if you're reading this you can probably relate.

Hiccups are extremely common, in that everybody

experiences them at some point. The fact that there seemed to be no widespread definitive solution to stop them lead me to the conclusion that, therefore, there was no sure fire way if ridding yourself of them, and that they were just something that had to be endured until they had run their natural course.

There are of course many 'cures' people have offered up over the years, however these invariably turn out to be nothing more than old wives tales. Some even appeared to work occasionally, but none consistently enough to be classed as credible remedies. The conclusion I came to was, in fact, that the only reason they ever worked is because I happened to try them at the point the hiccups were about to subside anyway.

One day I attended a friend's wedding, when a particularly severe bout of hiccups began. I was barely able to take a breath between spasms, let alone hold a conversation. This continued for nearly two hours before I was approached by another guest who assured me he could relieve my hiccups within seconds. Skeptical though I was, I was prepared to try anything to get back to normality and happily allowed him to try and work his magic.

Amazingly, true to his word, he achieved exactly as he'd promised and I was able to enjoy the rest of the reception hiccup-free. Despite the fact that I was still not completely convinced it had been his cure that had ceased my constant hiccups, I was actually kind of looking forward to my next bout to see if this really was the miracle cure I'd almost given up hope of finding.

It was only two days later I had the opportunity to put this method to the test once again. As soon as they began, I jumped at the chance to try it out immediately. I was both ecstatic and amazed to see it work again! I was now becoming more convinced that a hiccups cure was not just possible, but exceptionally easy.

I have since used this method countless times to cure hiccups, whether they be mine or somebody else's. The success rate has been 100%. This is not a placebo effect, a way of 'tricking' the mind; it is a genuine solution that works whether you believe it will or not.

What really surprises me about this method is that it is so little known. Almost everyone has heard some of the more common so called remedies out there: holding your breath for as long as you can, drinking a glass of water the wrong way round, or getting someone to make you jump being just some of these. But the truth is, although some people swear by one or more of these methods, they're generally unsuccessful and therefore cannot really be labelled as cures. Yet the one universal remedy that actually works appears to be known by very few. It was for this reason I decided to produce this short guide.

Please note that this cure is unlikely to work for cases of *accute* hiccups; that is, hiccups that go on for weeks or even months and are usually symptoms of a more serious illness.

2 WHAT ARE HICCUPS?

We all know what the effects of hiccups are: the unpredictable and irregular sudden intakes of breath and, ultimately, the internal pains that they bring with them. But what actually causes them?

There are actually several possible causes for hiccups, but by far the most common is irritation of the stomach, or the oesophagus (the tube that carries food to your stomach). For reasons that are not fully known, this can cause spasms in your diaphragm. The sudden intake of breath that subsequently occurs causes your glottis (the flap that separates your air and food tubes) to suddenly close, resulting in the 'hic' sound that we all know and love (although admittedly the word 'love' is probably the wrong word to use in this instance!).

There are no obvious evolutionary reasons for hiccups. They provide absolutely no known advantage to the human body and evolutionists can only speculate that they were once of some benefit in one of our evolutionary ancestors. This knowledge only serves to make their uncomfortable effect even more irritating!

Despite the knowledge that we do have of the processes that occur in the body when we have hiccups, and the conditions under which they are likely to occur, medical experts are still uncertain as to the *exact* mechanisms of hiccups.

In a practical sense, the following are some common causes of hiccups:

- Drinking too much alcohol
- Drastic and sudden changes of internal body temperature
- Swallowing too much air
- Eating food too quickly
- Smoking excessively

3 THE DEFINITIVE CURE FOR HICCUPS

What follows is the method that consistently works to cure hiccups. This is not an old wives tale, but something that has been proven time and again to remedy this annoyance once and for all.

This cure may sound absurd and shockingly simple, yet as long as you follow these simple instructions your hiccups will almost certainly subside within a few seconds.

As the exact mechanisms that cause and perpetuate hiccups are unknown, it is also uncertain why this method works as a cure, yet its effectiveness is indisputable.

The following steps will cure your hiccups:

1. Pour yourself a glass of water (although I have suggested water in this case, in actual fact any drinkable liquid can be used, however I would avoid fizzy drinks as these can actually cause

further stomach irritation and result in your hiccups starting again).

2. Plug your ears. By this, I simply mean to cover your ear canal so that no air can enter or exit your ears. Rather than sticking your fingers into your ear canal directly, the best way to do this is to push down on the flaps in front of your ear canals so they completely seal your ears.

3. While your ears are plugged, drink the glass of water, or as much of it as you can manage. This may seem like a difficult thing to do while you are also plugging your ears. You can get around this in two ways: either get somebody else to hold the glass of water for you, and slowly tip it into your mouth as you drink it; or plug your ears with your thumbs and use the rest of your fingers / palms to hold the glass as you drink (this can take a bit of practice to get used to!).

That really is it! As simple and obscure as this process seems, it really is the definitive cure for hiccups. You do not need to drink a massive amount of water to have the desired effect; a few sizeable gulps should do the job, as long as your ears are completely plugged while you are drinking it.

You may find that you hiccup while you are completing the exercise; this is completely normal. Just continue gulping until you can't manage any more. When you stop you may even experience one final hiccup before they disappear completely.

If in the unlikely event you try the above and it doesn't work the first time, repeat the steps again. It will almost certainly cure any bout of hiccups

4 SOME OTHER WELL KNOWN REMEDIES

For the sake of completeness I have decided to include some of the other well known remedies that have been suggested to me over the many years of my hiccup suffering. In the *highly unlikely* event that the above cure doesn't work for you, you may wish to try one or more of these.

Holding your breath

This is probably the best known suggestion for somebody who is suffering from hiccups. The idea is to hold your breath for as long as you possibly can. The hope is that by the time you finally have to succumb to breathing again your hiccups will be gone.

In actual fact, although I never found this method worked for me, some people do swear by it. While holding your breath, swallowing several times may further increase your chances of success.

Get somebody to make you jump

This is also a very widely publicised 'cure' for hiccups, however even if it does work it's actually extremely hard to do. Generally when you jump it is out of both fear and surprise. Deliberately implementing both of these conditions is not the easiest thing to do, particularly when you're already expecting it.

Suck on a lemon

Probably a slightly less well known cure is to suck on a slice of lemon. Adding sugar to the lemon may increase the effect. The bitterness is supposed to shock the body in a similar way to somebody making you jump (I've no idea how the sugar is supposed to help with this!). Though I've tried this several times in the past, it's never helped me in the slightest, yet a friend of mine has been using this as a cure for years.

A similar effect can be achieved by swallowing around half a teaspoon of salt. This probably isn't one of the more pleasant ways of attempting to stop your hiccups.

Gargle with water

Over the years, several people suggesting gargling with water as their ideal hiccups remedy. I've never seen this work. It's just difficult and very annoying, as you can end up choking when some of the water goes down the wrong hole!

Breathe into a paper bag

This is actually one of the slightly more credible sounding methods, as it helps to regulate your breathing in the same way as somebody who is hyper-ventilating may do. The problem is that there is rarely a paper bag around when you need one. I've never actually attempted this method so can't really comment too much on its efficacy.

.

5 A FINAL WORD

Congratulations! You now know how to cure your hiccups. If, like me, you've been a long sufferer of these inconvenient spasms you may already be experiencing the delight that I've felt ever since I first discovered this method. As sad as it may seem, I would not almost go so far as to say I enjoy getting hiccups purely for the experience of being able to cure them immediately.

Spread the word! There is no reason for this solution not to be more widely known. You may be surprised at the amount of appreciation you receive by curing others' hiccups; I've received many a free pint for this simple but handy piece of advice.

Here's to the end of your suffering!

ACKNOWLEDGEMENTS

I would like to acknowledge John Ferriman. Without my chance meeting with John at Rosie and Paul's wedding I may never have learned about this wonderful remedy.

ABOUT THE AUTHOR

Gareth Forman is a web designer and freelance journalist, who lives with his wife and three children in Leicestershire, England. He has been happily hiccup-free for more than four years now.